Sorin Baschir
Radmila- Anca Bugari

Phototherapy in the treatment of allergic rhinitis

AF135940

Sorin Baschir
Radmila- Anca Bugari

Phototherapy in the treatment of allergic rhinitis

LAP LAMBERT Academic Publishing

Impressum / Imprint

Bibliografische Information der Deutschen Nationalbibliothek: Die Deutsche Nationalbibliothek verzeichnet diese Publikation in der Deutschen Nationalbibliografie; detaillierte bibliografische Daten sind im Internet über http://dnb.d-nb.de abrufbar.
Alle in diesem Buch genannten Marken und Produktnamen unterliegen warenzeichen-, marken- oder patentrechtlichem Schutz bzw. sind Warenzeichen oder eingetragene Warenzeichen der jeweiligen Inhaber. Die Wiedergabe von Marken, Produktnamen, Gebrauchsnamen, Handelsnamen, Warenbezeichnungen u.s.w. in diesem Werk berechtigt auch ohne besondere Kennzeichnung nicht zu der Annahme, dass solche Namen im Sinne der Warenzeichen- und Markenschutzgesetzgebung als frei zu betrachten wären und daher von jedermann benutzt werden dürften.

Bibliographic information published by the Deutsche Nationalbibliothek: The Deutsche Nationalbibliothek lists this publication in the Deutsche Nationalbibliografie; detailed bibliographic data are available in the Internet at http://dnb.d-nb.de.
Any brand names and product names mentioned in this book are subject to trademark, brand or patent protection and are trademarks or registered trademarks of their respective holders. The use of brand names, product names, common names, trade names, product descriptions etc. even without a particular marking in this works is in no way to be construed to mean that such names may be regarded as unrestricted in respect of trademark and brand protection legislation and could thus be used by anyone.

Coverbild / Cover image: www.ingimage.com

Verlag / Publisher:
LAP LAMBERT Academic Publishing
ist ein Imprint der / is a trademark of
OmniScriptum GmbH & Co. KG
Heinrich-Böcking-Str. 6-8, 66121 Saarbrücken, Deutschland / Germany
Email: info@lap-publishing.com

Herstellung: siehe letzte Seite /
Printed at: see last page
ISBN: 978-3-659-54453-8

Contents

Objectives and rationale for the study

The main objective of the study is to prove the effectiveness, tolerability and safety of rhinophototherapy as an alternative method in the treatment of allergic rhinitis, and its superiority first over placebo, then over classic medication – antihistamines administered generally or corticoids administered locally.

There are numerous general objectives, as well as numerous reasons why we decided to conduct this study, which we shall detail below.

Allergic rhinitis is defined clinically as a symptomatic "disorder" of the nasal mucosa, caused by an inflammation induced by immunoglobulin E (IgE), following exposure to respiratory allergens; symptoms of allergic rhinitis include nasal obstruction, sneezing in volleys and aqueous rhinorrhea; these symptoms compose the major symptomatological triad, while some minor symptoms include: ocular symptoms (pruritus, lacrimation), the posterior drainage of secretions and, last but not least, general symptoms affecting the patient's social life.

This last decade has seen an exponential increase in cases of allergic rhinitis, an issue which can be found across the European continent and which, in the area targeted by our study, is found in about 20-25% of the total population; the study we propose refers to four counties in the west of Romania - Arad, Timiş, Bihor, Satu Mare – and to the corresponding cross-border area in Hungary; this geographic area totals some 4 million inhabitants – 2,200,000 in the Romanian counties and 1,800,000 in similar areas from Hungary.

The methodology of this study was elaborated after lengthy searches, which entailed: the study of the literature, the personal experience of the physicians involved – otorhinolaryngologists, allergologists, pulmonologists, pediatricians, family physicians –, meetings and consultations with colleagues of similar specialties in Hungary, resulting in the unanimously accepted conclusion that allergic rhinitis has become a general health issue (the very high percentage, 20-25% of the population, which, however, seems to be underestimated, as many patients do not recognize allergic rhinitis and do not go see a doctor). Likewise, by studying recent statistics, we observed that allergic rhinitis has become a very frequent, top reason for primary visits to medical practices; the illness is not severe or life-threatening, but it has become particularly important because it affects the patients' quality of life, wellbeing, and social life – which in turn affects academic performance and work productivity. Another element of severity in this illness is represented by the possible association, very common in practice, with other pathological states, the first of which is asthma, then sinusitis, otitis media, nasal polyps and lower respiratory tract infection.

In our study we used the classification proposed by ARIA - Allergic Rhinitis and Impact on Asthma - in which allergic rhinitis is classified, according to its duration and severity, into:

-           intermittent allergic rhinitis - symptoms last for less than four days per week and less than four weeks overall
-           persistent allergic rhinitis - symptoms last for more than four days per week and more than four weeks overall.

According to its severity, rhinitis can be divided into:
- mild form – in which the patient does not experience sleep disturbances, day-to-day activity is not disrupted, and academic/workplace performance is normal
- moderate or severe form – in which the patient experiences impairment in sleep, day-to-day activity, academic performance, etc

In the study we have undertaken we agreed that it is more important, for reasons of scientific accuracy and rigorousness, to use the term of clinically, endoscopically and especially allergologically confirmed allergic rhinitis, its clinical form – seasonal (intermittent) or perennial (persistent) – being of lesser importance, and to test, as accurately as possible, the efficiency of various therapeutic methods.

Another important reason for starting this study was the poor outcome obtained by drug therapy in the treatment of allergic rhinitis, as all therapeutic attempts have had a high percentage of failure – both general and/or local therapy, a percentage which, according to some authors, might even go as far as exceed 50%.

Yet another very important reason is the high cost of drug therapy, the lengthy treatment period required to obtain favorable results, ranging from two to three weeks, as well as the fact that the patient is bound by the administration of a drug.

Studying allergic rhinitis led us to the conclusion that it has become a general health issue and even a social one, given its high frequency in the two cross-border regions we studied: since 4,000,000 inhabitants live in the region included in the study, and the percentage of allergic rhinitis is estimated at 20% (although we believe it to be greater), this means that 800,000 to 1,000,000 people suffers from allergic rhinitis, which is a very large number.

Another issue that worries and concerns us is the decrease in the age threshold for allergic rhinitis, with the onset of the disorder found at increasingly younger ages, where drug treatment is difficult to administer, often even contraindicated, with unfavorable therapeutic outcomes.

Consequently, we wish to review some of the most important objectives and motives for the study of rhinophototherapy as an alternative method to the classic treatment of allergic rhinitis:

        - the main objective is to study phototherapy in the treatment of allergic rhinitis, by comparing it to classic drug treatment and placebo therapy

- allergic rhinitis has become a global health issue given the frequency of this disorder – approximately 1,000,000 Romanian and Hungarian inhabitants in the studied area

-the healthcare costs for these patients are very high, which is why it is important to find a more efficient and, at the same time, less expensive method

-drug therapy for allergic rhinitis has a high percentage of failure

- allergic rhinitis is not life-threatening, but it is often associated with numerous diseases whose onset it might favor: asthma, rhinosinusitis, otitis media, repeated lower respiratory tract infection

- allergic rhinitis affects the patients' quality of life, their social life, academic performance and work productivity

- through our joint effort we wish to discover an efficient, safe, inexpensive therapeutic method, with no significant side effects, which might improve the health state and quality of life of our patients, both Romanian and Hungarian, as disease knows no boundaries or differences among us.

Allergic rhinitis

1. Symptoms

Most of the times, the patient experiences the following symptoms:

- Intense, violent sneezing "in volleys"
- Watery nasal secretion
- Partial/ total bilateral nasal obstruction
- Nasal pruritus often associated, as is conjunctivitis with excessive tearing, ocular pruritus, foreign body sensation in the eyelids.

The symptomatic profile of patients afflicted by perennial rhinitis is different from that of seasonal allergic rhinitis:
- more frequent in **perennial rhinitis**:
  - nasal obstruction
  - rhinorrhea
- more frequent in **seasonal allergic rhinitis**:
  - pruritus
  - sneezing

2.Possibly associated symptoms:

- Headache, tension in the sinuses
- Fatigue, irritability and insomnia, when AR lasts for several days or weeks.
- Mouth breathing
- Hyposmia
- Eustachian tube dysfunction, sensation of pressure in the ear or hearing impairment
- Dark circles around the eyes
- Frequent nose rubbing with the palm facing up (allergic "salute") - children
- Cough - dry at first, then it may become productive
- Pruritus of the palate
- Conjunctival irritation with pruritus and lacrimation

3.Comorbidities:

- Asthma: when bronchial inflammation also occurs
- Chronic pharyngitis
- Chronic seromucous otitis
- Chronic sinusitis
- Allergic conjunctivitis
- Histamine release in very large amounts may lead to anaphylaxis.

Allergies are an attribute of subjects with genetic predisposition for atopy, their evolution frequently assuming the picture known as "allergic march": food allergies since the very first months of life, atopic dermatitis, and later allergic rhinitis and asthma, with sensitization to inhaled allergens.

4.Positive diagnosis:

Allergic rhinitis should be suspected after detailed case history and can be confirmed by skin testing for inhaled allergens and/or serological testing.

1) Case history and symptomatology:

It is based on the same principles as in any other disorder, being often indicative for identifying the allergen.
Case history: - for how long the symptoms have been present,
- family and collateral history,
- work and life conditions (presence of house pets, dietary habits, changes in symptoms during holidays etc.)

A. Pollen allergy: it is easy to diagnose due to its characteristic periodicity.The onset is in childhood or adolescence, while symptoms appear each year, with varying intensity. After the age of 50, allergic rhinoconjunctivitis due to pollen improves considerably.
Symptoms are manifested characteristically in the open air, especially during sunny days. Nasal congestion is frequent, more accentuated in the evening and at night.
Ocular pruritus and congestion are constant, and rubbing accentuates them (vicious circle). Some patients complain of pharyangeal and otic pruritus, fatigue, adynamia, headache and anorexia. About 20% of patients can associate asthma attacks.
The severity of symptoms depends on the concentration of pollen in the atmosphere: higher on sunny, dry days and lower on damp, cold ones.

B. Allergy to house dust mites(Dermatophagoides) leads to persistent symptoms, being exacerbated, in some older houses, while making the bed or during cleaning. Symptoms are generally identical to seasonal rhinitis, but ocular pruritus is rarer and nasal congestion more manifest. Although severity varies, AR to mites is a year-round nuisance.

C. Symptoms triggered by inhaling pet (dog and cat) allergens are permanent, but more severe, improved when outside of the house (with dogs or cats).

D. Occupational allergens cause the exacerbation of symptoms at work and improvement during weekends or holidays.

E. Mold allergy is manifested perennially, with seasonal exacerbation, especially in very damp places. Sometimes, people who are allergic to inhaled fungi may have symptoms after ingesting foods that ferment with molds (wine, beer, pressed cheese).

- Some patients predominantly experience sneezing and aqueous rhinorrhea, also known as "sneezers and runners"
- Other patients predominantly experience nasal congestion and mucous secretions – "blockers"

For a complete evaluation the patient must mention his/her age at the onset of the disease, the evolution of symptoms throughout the years, the influence of home changes, the nature of the workplace, the presence of allergic disorders in the patient's family, etc. It is important to identify weekly or seasonal variations of symptoms. The severity of symptoms, assessed by means of their duration and frequency, dictate the correct classification of the degree of severity and the correct therapeutic attitude.

2) Objective examination

- Children often make grimaces or scratch their nose – "allergic salute", which leads to the formation of transversal folds in the lower third of the nose.
- If obstruction is severe: mouth breathing, predisposing to high arched palate and dental modifications, with patients having infra orbital dark circles.
- Anterior rhinoscopy reveals violaceous edema of the nasal mucosa.
  Objective examination should be complemented with eye, skin and lung examination.

3) Skin allergy testing:

Skin testing, associated with correct case history and objective examination, are often sufficient to establish the diagnosis. In recent years, allergological diagnosis has been improved by allergen standardization and the availability of extracts for most inhaled allergens.

The PRICK method is the most useful allergological examination. The limit of positivity is 3mm for the papule if the control is negative. The reaction is read at 15 min. There is a good correlation of the prick test with allergic symptoms and an easier distinction of positive tests from negative ones. Before testing, antihistamines must be stopped for a while, depending on their half-life.

A positive result signifies the presence of specific IgE antibodies to that allergen, but does not necessarily certify the diagnosis of allergic disease. About 25% of young people have positive tests, but only 15% develop symptoms, while the rest are at risk of becoming symptomatic.

The diagnosis of persistent allergic rhinitis is based on allergy history and skin testing, rather than on the examination of the nose.

4) RAST – Radioallergosorbent test:

A blood sample is harvested and tested for immunoglobulins E. This test is more expensive than the skin test, the results are available after about a week and can yield a false-positive response.

5) Nasal cytology (nasal smear):

It measures the number of eosinophils, which are present in large amounts in the nasal mucosa of allergic people. The test can be used to confirm allergic rhinitis and to differentiate infectious from non-infectious and eosinophilic from non-eosinophilic rhinitis. The presence of eosinophils in a percentage higher than 10% is indicative of allergic rhinitis or eosinophilic non-allergic rhinitis. In acute infections, neutrophils are predominant in the nasal secretion

6) Nasal endoscopy

It is required in all cases of chronic rhinitis and sinusitis. In allergic rhinitis the nasal mucosa is swollen, pale blue in color, covered in clear secretions. In viral infections, in smokers and in cases of local decongestant abuse, the mucosa is red.

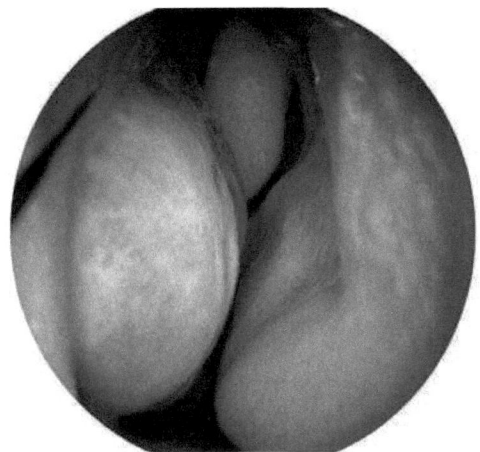

7) Computerized tomography:

It is the examination of choice in detecting anatomic anomalies, the nasal polyps of sinusitis. It is indicated in selected cases: with severe chronic symptoms to rule out malignity and before surgical intervention. Diagnostic input is maximal in detecting ethmoidal sinusitis.

8) Rhinomanometry:

It is a technique which measures the flow of air in the nose. The test provides an estimation of nasal congestion or obstruction due to AR, nasal polyps and other causes. Rhinomanometry is generally used in research. Rhinomanometry is an objective method of study which measures the permeability of nostrils, by evaluating resistance to air flow and recording the *pressure-flow* and *area-distance* curves.

Rhinomanometry clasification:

- Active anterior rhinomanometry
- Posterior rhinomanometry
- Passive anterior rhinomanometry
- Acoustic rhinomanometry

Differential diagnosis:

AR diagnosis is complicated, exceeding the boundaries of ENT and overlapping with allergological diagnosis, and is made with:

- **Mechanic or structural factors:**

  - Foreign bodies
  - Nasal septum deviation
  - Ostiomeatal anomalies
  - Adenoid hypertrophy
  - Nasal polyps
  - Benign and malignant tumors

- **Acute and chronic infections:**

  - Viral
  - Bacterial
  - Mycotic

- **Immunologic diseases:**

- Wegener's granulomatosis
- sarcoidosis
- systemic lupus erythematosus
- Sjögren's syndrome
- amyloidosis
- rhinosclerom

- **Various:**

- Perennial eosinophilic rhinitis
- Hormonal rhinitis
- Drug-induced rhinitis
- Occupational rhinitis
- Atrophic rhinitis
- Ciliary defects
- Cerebrospinal rhinorrhea

Symptoms	Allergic rhinitis	Vasomotor instability	Non-allergic rhinitis with eosinophilia syndrome	Drug-induced rhinitis	Structural rhinitis	Rhinosinusitis	Nasal polyps
Cause/mechanisms	...ergy	Vascular	Unknown	Inappropriate medication	Septum deviation	Infection	Eosinophilic inflammation
Sneezing and pruritus	+++	-	++++	-	-	-	-
Rhinorrhea	+++	+/-	++++	-	-	Purulence	+
Obstruction	++	++++	+/-	+++	+++	++	++++
Post-nasal drip	+	++++	+/-	-	-	+++	++
Seasonal variations	Seasonal or perennial	Perennial	Perennial	Perennial	Perennial	Perennial	Perennial
Eosinophils in nasal secretion	+	-	+	-	-	-	+
Skin tests	Positive	Negative	Negative	Negative	Negative	Negative	Negative
Age of onset	Childhood	Adulthood	Any age	Adulthood	Any age	Any age	Adulthood
Associated factors	Atopy in the family, pale mucosa	Pregnancy, thyroid disease	Pale mucosa	Adm. of decongestant drops, antihypertensive drugs	Unilateral obstruction, history of nasal trauma	Associated respiratory infection	Aspirin sensitivity

++++=marked +++=moderate ++=mild +/-=questionable -=absent

DIFFERENTIAL DIAGNOSIS OF RHINITIS (modified according to Silvin R.G)

Complcations of allergic rhinitis:

The most frequent complications of AR are due to the fact that the common element is ATOPY.

Owing to the contiguity of nasal mucosa with the mucosa of paranasal sinuses, the rhinopharynx and the middle ear, AR, especially the persistent type, is frequently complicated by otitis media and sinusitis:

- **Otitis media** is most common in children. Nasal mucosa edema and the excess of secretions may obstruct the Eustachian tube, causing serous otitis media.
- **Acute sinusitis** – another complication of AR is clinically suggested by the persistence of symptoms (nasal obstruction, rhinorrhea – mucous at first then purulent, headache) for more than 10 days, or the aggravation of these symptoms. Allergic rhinitis is only complicated by sinusitis in cases of persistent nasal congestion, with the obstruction of sinus ostia by the accumulation of secretions, with bacterial infection potential. Most frequently involved are maxillary and ethmoidal sinuses. Pathogenic bacteria most frequently involved are Streptococcus pneumoniae, H. influenza and M. catarrhalis.
- **Chronic sinusitis** is the inflammation of paranasal sinuses for a period longer than 3 months. It is more common in adults and manifested by rhinorrhea, the rhinopharyngeal drainage of nasal secretions, which can induce persistent, predominantly nocturnal cough, headache, halitosis, chronic nasal obstruction and treatment-resistant asthma. Chronic sinusitis may also be caused by anaerobic bacteria: Peptostreptococcus, Corynebacterium. The diagnosis of certainty is radiological (CT).
- **Allergic or infectious conjunctivitis**
- **Nasal polyps** (with partial or total obstruction), with the exacerbation of asthma, often coexistent.
- **Infections of the respiratory tract:** asthma, chronic pharyngolaryngitis

Allergic rhinitis therapeutic principles

The therapeutic treatment plan comprises:

1. **Preventive measures**:

Reduce exposure to the incriminated allergen(s). For patients suffering from AR with IgE-mediated sensitization to mites, and especially pollens, the allergologist can recommend, in some situations, a number of specific precautions linked to the possible cross-reactivity between airborne allergens and certain food allergens. In addition, it is recommended to avoid exposure to non-specific irradiants, especially tobacco smoke.

2. **Pharmacological treatment**:

It depends on the degree of severity of AR, as well as on the patient's individual symptoms. The following drugs are commonly employed:
- o H1 antihistamines,
- o intranasal corticosteroids,
- o (sometimes) systemic corticosteroids,
- o nasal decongestants,
- o chromones
- o nasal anticholinergics,
- o antileukotrienes (preferred in the case of patients with coexisting asthma)

3. **Immunotherapy:**

With allergenic vaccines: it is recommended in patients suffering from rhinitis with IgE-mediated mechanism, demonstrated in positive skin allergy testing and/or specific serum IgE. The benefit/risk ratio must be taken into consideration. It is prescribed by the allergologist to improve symptoms in patients with sensitization to mites or pollens. The administration of immunotherapy for 3-4 years can induce prolonged symptom remission, and in children it can reduce the probability of developing asthma. There are vaccines administered by subcutaneous, sublingual or intranasal injection.

4.**Alternative therapies**:

a) Rhinolight is the newest therapeutic method, applied locally, with the advantage of no systemic side effects that are possible in the case of drug therapy
   - This therapy has a strong immunosuppressive effect and is able to inhibit hypersensitivity reactions of the allergic mucosa

- The application of rhinophototherapy significantly reduces nasal obstruction, anterior and posterior rhinorrhea, while also acting on other symptoms of AR
- Results are immediate and visible
- Rhinophototherapy is an alternative to antihistamine drug therapy – either as single therapy, or as a supplement to drug therapy.

b) Phythotherapy.

Skin prick test and specific Ig-E dosage:

Allergic rhinitis is clinically defined as a symptomatic "disorder" emerging in the nose and induced by exposure to allergens, whose intimate mechanism is represented by IgE-mediated inflammation in the nasal mucosa (1).

Case history, which is of primordial importance, and physical examination are not sufficient to differentiate between allergic and non-allergic rhinitis, they must be complemented by paraclinical investigations (2).

Skin allergy tests represent a specific investigation in allergology, with a key contribution in identifying the allergen, provided the results are corroborated with history data (3).

Skin allergy tests can be run for any patient suspected of allergic rhinitis, even children under one year (4); it is, however necessary, to use the right allergens according to the patient's age and to the period of the year in which the symptoms appear.

Prick-testing, updated since 1970 by Pepys and utilized mostly in Europe, consists of pricking the skin on the forearm or back with one drop of allergen solution in glycerin, initially deposited in these areas, while the needle does not penetrate the dermis. (5).

Allergenic extracts for prick tests are highly stable extracts (1-2 years), whose stability is given by the content of 50% glycerol extracts or by human serum albumin – in the case of lyophilized allergenic extracts.

An important element for diagnosis is the inoculated amount of allergen, which in turn depends on the potency of the extract. The potency of the extract is expressed in units that are specific to the companies which prepare these allergenic extracts. Recently, in Europe, standardization was imposed through biological methods based on the medium reactivity to allergens of some groups of tested allergic patients, which has allowed the obtainment of positive tests, with a 5-8 mm average of papule diameters in prick-tests (6). Currently, there is standardization through biological methods applying to some extracts for the main pneumo-allergens (house dust and mites, pollens, animal skin products – dog, cat, rabbit, horse, guinea pig –, alternaria, cladosporium etc.

As regards the **technique used** in prick-testing, there are two methods, namely: a drop of the allergen solution is initially deposited on the skin of the forearm or back, in a free area and in the control one, then we proceed to:

a) utilize a syringe needle (for hypodermic or intradermal injection), which is applied to the epidermal layer parallel to the skin, after having passed through the drop of allergen or control solution, then pulled out, by slightly raising the skin, without causing local bleeding. The surplus of allergen or control solution will subsequently be wiped off.

b) utilize standardized needles such as: the Morrow-Brown needle, the Osterballe needle or the Stallerprick needle, needles which prevent the exaggerate penetration of the epidermis, being outfitted with a 1mm tip, flanked by two "shoulders" which dictate pricking depth. This technique entails two rules, namely: the needle will be held perpendicularly to the skin, so that the pricking angle would be 90 degrees, and the pricking pressure would be constantly applied for one second (7).

Whatever needle is utilized, the distance between two pricks should be 2 cm, pricking depth should be around 1mm, and allergens drops should not mix. We shall use one needle for one test and one needle kit for one patient, so as to avoid the risk of "allergen contamination".

As for the number of prick tests, it will be established according to thorough allergological history.

Interpreting results.

A *positive test* will be a papule of a diameter of up to 3 mm, but if the diameter of the papule for the control solution is smaller than 2 mm, a papule measuring 2 mm in diameter will also be accepted as positive reaction. It is preferable to record the result of testing in mm, and mention the appearance of pseudopodia or local pruritus, or any other syndrome reaction (6, 7).

The diagnostic value of prick testing in the case of positive results, especially for papule diameters of over 5 mm, is significant, in correlation with clinical data, as that allergen can be incriminated in the appearance of clinical symptoms (5, 6, 7). In clinical practice, most of the times there is a major etiological involvement from 1-2 allergens and latent (subclinical) allergy to other allergens which is not manifested during test positivization, but which can manifest itself clinically over the following months, or even years, in those patients. Bousquet believes that latent allergens are only involved in the emergence of allergic rhinitis in cases where their concentration is extremely high.

EAACI established the following as essential elements in performing skin testing with diagnostic values and in the incrimination of an allergen in the etiology of the disease:

    a) the quality of the extract: constant biological activity and sufficient potency

    b) the same technique used in testing (8).

The limits of skin testing are linked to: the nature of the allergen, factors modifying skin reactivity: age, comorbidity, the season when the testing occurs, drugs administered prior to testing.

It is accepted that skin tests are feasible and interpretable since the age of 3 months and that they are diminished in old age.

The site of skin testing in the diagnostic algorithm of the allergic etiology of rhinitis is extremely important.

In vitro dosage of specific IgE is one of the criteria for diagnosing immediate hypersensitivity. In allergic rhinitis, specific IgE are found in increased amounts in nasal secretions, being largely synthesized locally (9). IgE level, generally greatly decreased compared to other immunoglobulins, increases in patients with type I allergic reaction, this antibody being responsible for immediate hypersensitivity reactions (10).

Comparisons regarding the diagnostic value of skin testing in relation to the dosage of specific IgE

In vitro dosage of specific serum IgE has a few inconveniences, as well as some advantages compared to skin testing.

Advantages of skin testing over serum IgE dosage:
- simplicity, expedience, lower costs.
- It can be used for several allergens
- A more faithful parallel can be drawn between its severity and clinical evolution
- It may complement and detail the positive result obtained at the Phadia-top screening (multi-RAST detecting "the allergy state" of the patient).

Advantages of serum IgE dosage over skin testing:
- It is not influenced by previous treatments
- It can be performed for patients with extended dermatoses
- It can detect the allergy state in infants and the elderly, where skin testing yields results that are difficult to interpret.

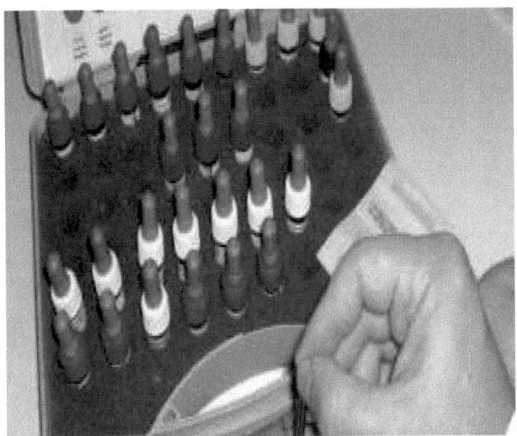

Conclusion

Allergic rhinitis, with IgE mediated hypersensitivity to airborne allergens, has an important prevalence. People in the 21-30 age group was most frequently assigned the diagnosis of allergic rhinitis, followed by the 31-40 group, which means young adults are the most affected. The number of cases of allergic rhinitis decreases with age. Airborne allergens most frequently incriminated in IgE-mediated hypersensitivity in allergic rhinitis are mites and pollens, followed, in decreasing order of frequency, by animal epithelia and molds. Among house dust mites, *Dermatophagoides pteronyssinus* and *Dermatophagoides farinae* have been incriminated in an almost equal proportion. Among pollens, the airborne allergen most frequently incriminated in causing allergic rhinitis symptoms is grass pollen, which in our country pollinates during the months of May-July. Among animal epithelia, most cases of IgE- mediated hypersensitivity are to cat epithelia.

Serological investigations in allergology

Eligible methods in the paraclinical diagnosis of allergic diseases are the following (1)
- Total serum IgE dosage
- Specific IgE dosage
- Specific IgG dosage
- ECP (eosinophil cationic protein) dosage
- Leukotriene dosage
- Measuring the histamine release from mast cells

The first two methods are utilized in current clinical practice, whereas the others have a role in research.

Total serum IgE.
The determination of total serum IgE is today seen as an obsolete method, as it has low sensitivity (12%), false negative cases being numerous (1). In a study conducted in Germany and including 325 adult patients, the comparison of clinical data with IgE levels has yielded the following results (values above 100 kU/l are considered positive):

IgE level (kU/l)	Allergic patients	Non-allergic patients
0-25	25	20
25-50	40	20
50-100	25	10
100-200	70	10
> 200	100	5

For this reason, the determination of total IgE is not deemed useful in the diagnosis of respiratory allergies, however, an increased IgE level can be a prognostic indicator in children with atopic dermatitis, and a possible indicator of atopic disease progression towards multi-organic locations (2,3,4).

Specific IgE
The determination of specific IgE is today regarded as the standard *in vitro* diagnostic method in allergology. The advantages of this method are multiple:
- increased sensitivity and specificity, similar to skin testing
- repeatability, with a smaller source of error that in the case of skin tests
- it can be performed in cases when skin testing is contraindicated (acute exacerbation of atopic diseases, medication, pregnancy etc.)
- it is less traumatic than other diagnostic methods, such as the intracutaneous test, while also enabling the determination of sensitivity to many allergens during a single intervention, which is of particular importance for children
- it is an accurate, quantifiable method for monitoring the efficiency of specific immunotherapy.

With all these advantages, it must be underlined that any *in vitro* determination highlights sensitivity to allergens, and cannot establish all by itself the diagnosis of atopic disease - this being the task of an allergologist.

The methods for determining specific IgE are usually semi-quantitative. The fact that there are no standardized units of measurement, accepted by international consensus, means that the results of the different methods to determine specific IgE are only comparable within the same system (for example, results obtained in the Pharmacia CAP system are not comparable to those in the AllergyScreen system).

The AllergyScreen technique is a semi-quantitative imunoblotting method and has the following phases:

- serum is incubated on a slide
- biotinylated anti-IgE antibodies are added
- streptavidin is coupled to biotin molecules
- reaction with NBT, resulting in the formation of a linear precipitation. The intensity of this staining is proportional to the amount of specific IgE in the patient's serum. Results are read using an optical camera, represented graphically and presented to the patient in printed form.

Rhinomanometry

Nasal obstruction is one of the main symptoms of allergic rhinitis, which is why its measurement using objective methods is important in managing AR diagnosis.

Rhinomanometry is an objective study method which measures nostril permeability by evaluating resistance to air flow while recording the pressure-flow and area-distance curves.

Rhinomanometry offers objective and quantitative indications on nasal permeability, being dependent on two parameters:
- Differential pressure Δp: it is the difference between the air pressure measured in the mask at the level of nasal vestibules and the inspiratory and expiratory pressure at the level of the choanae, expressed in Pa.
- Flow rate V: it represents the volume of air passing through the nostrils in the time unit, measured in cm^3/s

By simultaneously measuring differential pressure and flow rate, a flow rate/pressure curve is obtained, which represents the nasal pressure curve.

- Very important nasal obstruction = 0 to 500 cm^3/s
- Average nasal obstruction = 500 to 700 cm^3/s
- Less important nasal obstruction = 700 to 870 cm^3/s
- Insignificant nasal obstruction = over 870 cm^3/s

Rhinomanometry is a complementary method for examining nasal permeability, which allows measuring the transversal section in different areas of the nose, depending on distance. It is currently used across the world and its indications are well established:
1. in determining normal values in the initial situation for men and women
2. quantifying the increase in normal values after vasoconstriction
3. the study of differences between normal values in men and women
4. the sensitivity and specificity of rhinomanometry in measuring nasal obstruction
5. detecting anatomic nasal anomalies
6. the consistency between nasal symptoms and rhinomanometric values

Normal values in men:
- 0.77cm^2 at 0.18cm from the nostrils

- 0.56cm^2 at 1.87cm from the nostrils
Normal values in women:
- 0.55cm^2 at 0.26cm from the nostrils
- 0.47cm^2 at 1.83cm from the nostrils

Vasoconstriction causes an increase in the total nasal diameter, on average in the first 5 cm, by 30%. The area most affected by growth is the transversal section at 4 cm from the nostril, with growth averaging 55% in men and 39% in women.

Likewise, rhinomanometric values are proportional to the height of each person, being higher in taller people.

Clasification

- Active anterior rhinomanometry
- Posterior rhinomanometry
- Passive anterior rhinomanometry
- Acoustic rhinomanometry

Acoustic rhinomanometry:

➢ A relatively new method

➢ Consists of the analysis of a pulsatile sound wave transmitted along the nasal respiratory tract, which is then reflected back, due to changes in the transversal section area of the nasal cavity

➢ If the section area of nostrils is over 0.05 cm^2, acoustic rhinomanometry can be used (below 0.05 cm^2 it becomes impossible).

➢ Advantages of the method:
  - Fast and efficient, non-invasive screening
  - It can be performed in children
  - Records are kept in the database, using subsequent comparison

➢ The reflected sound passes through a microphone into a computer, where it is processed and presented as a graph: nasal section surface / distance

➢ The patient is requested to perform voluntary apnea

➢ Transnasal air flow is measured as air volume expressed in liters/minute

➢ The method can be used for any nostril with a section area > 0.05 cm^2

➢ This test is used in:

- Direct assessment of nasal obstruction in AR, nasal polyps, tumors, other space-occupying masses
- Assessment of the nasal function before and after decongestion
- Pre- and post-operative objective control in the surgery of septum deviation, cartilages and bones of the nasal pyramid

Conclusions:

It is an **objective method** which:

- provides a reproducible, quantifiable evaluation of nasal obstruction
- is easy to perform
- records can be used to evaluate post-therapy results.

Phototherapy

Definition

The term *phototherapy* denotes the use of light for therapeutic or preventive purposes (1). In the strict sense of the term, phototherapy would only include the use of electromagnetic waves in the visible spectrum (wavelengths ranging from 400 to 760 nm), but, in a broader sense, it is accepted to include procedures which apply ultraviolet or infrared waves, as well as those which apply photosensitizing agents: photochemotherapy, as well as photodynamic treatment.

The source of light can be natural (Sun - heliotherapy) or artificial.

Brief history

The Sun was worshipped by the majority of ancient civilizations. The shape of the solar disk was a symbol of the Universe and the Creator, and the red color of the Sun symbolized life (2, 3).

The use of sun baths by the Greeks and Romans is well documented (1).

In ancient China, heliotherapy was introduced by Taoists in the first century AD as an immortalization technique by capturing the vital energy (Qi) of the Sun. Another "heliotherapy" technique during the Tang dynasty consisted of morning exposure to sun rays, holding a ticket in one's right hand, on which the Sun sign was painted, surrounded by a red square. After the ritual, the irradiated ticket was soaked in water and swallowed, thus introducing a part of the essence of Sun into the body (1).

In medieval Europe, the first pharmacopeia in English, *"Rosa Medicinae"*, from the 15th century, comprises the use of red light (obtained by burning a candle) to prevent suppuration and pruritus in variolic skin lesions (1).

Applications of light based on cultic reasons were followed by scientific research regarding the nature and biological effects of solar light. Thus, Newton observed the phenomenon of refraction through a prism: the decomposition of monochrome light into the colors of the spectrum (1666); Christian Huygens (1678) elaborated the theory of the nature of light as a wave; Sir Frederic Herschel (1800) and Johann Ritter (1801) described the infrared and ultraviolet components of solar light (1). The microbicidal effect of the ultraviolet component of solar light was demonstrated in 1877 by Arthur Downes and Thomas Blunt (Anglia), who laid the bases for subsequent research in physiology and physiopathology regarding the biological effects of sun rays on the human body (1).

The pioneer of modern phototherapy was Niels Finsen, a winner of the Nobel Prize. After prior publications regarding the prevention of suppuration and pruritus in variolic lesions ("Rosa Medicinae" being unknown to him), he demonstrated the bactericidal effect of ultraviolet light (obtained from sunlight by applying filters which excluded wave lengths in the visible and infrared spectrum) on Koch's bacillum in lupus vulgaris lesions. Subsequently, sun light was replaced with lamps running on mercury vapors.

Soon, UV phototherapy was widely used to treat the consequences of the industrial revolution in cities of northern Europe, namely tuberculosis and rickets. Later, the improvement of living conditions and the introduction of anti-tuberculosis and anti-rickets drug treatments, along with the discovery of the carcinogenic effects of UV radiation, diminished their scope of use in the treatment of inflammatory skin diseases, often associated with photosensitizing agents (photochemotherapy). The therapeutic use of visible light evolved in parallel to that of UV light, its main indication becoming the treatment of neonatal jaundice.

Biological effects

a) visible light

The main indication of visible-light phototherapy is the treatment of neonatal jaundice. The therapeutic effect of light on jaundice was discovered based on the observation of oxidative transformation of serum bilirubin into biliverdin in a sample of blood accidentally put under light: bilirubin was decomposed into colorless products. At the same time, a nurse observed the improvement of neonatal jaundice in the case of exposure to sun rays of some parts of the body, while the unexposed surface remained jaundiced. The *in vitro* and *in vivo* findings led to idea that the exposure of teguments to the effect of blue sun rays improves neonatal jaundice by decreasing the concentration of serum bilirubin. It was subsequently found that, in fact, the decrease in the level of bilirubin is due, to a small extent, to the slow photodegradation into biliverdin; the essential reaction is that of rapid photochemical transformation of bilirubin into conformational isomers which will be conjugated in the liver and excreted with the bile. Likewise, it was found that white artificial light is as efficient as the blue form, but much cheaper, which is why the large-scale use of this type of phototherapy is indicated (1).

Colored light found its main indications in dermatological diseases: red and blue light are applied in the treatment of acne vulgaris (4, 5), and red light-emitting diodes (LED), applied to healthy people, have the effect of increasing fibroblastic activity (with no signs of inflammation) and increasing the number of Th-1 lymphocytes and, more markedly, Th-2 cells (6) in the skin.

There have also been interesting results obtained with white light in various neurological and psychiatric disorders: thus, there have been reports of significant improvements of chronic tension-type headache, moderate improvements of migraine in children (7), improvements in depressive and bipolar disorders (8), as well as the post-phototherapy improvement in the circadian rhythm sleep disorder (9).

b) ultraviolet light

Radiation in the ultraviolet spectrum of short (UVB 310-330 nm) or long (UVA 340-400 nm) wavelength has current therapeutic applications, as mentioned above, mostly in the area of dermatological disorders. Thus, UVA rays are used in the treatment of localized sclerodermia, systemic lupus erythematosus and polymorphous photodermatiosis (10), and in association with 8-methoxypsoralen (PUVA) it is applied in the treatment of atopic dermatitis and chronic and acute graft-versus-host reaction of the skin (11). The biological background of the anti-inflammatory action of UVA light can be: decreased expression of interferon gamma, induced apoptosis in infiltrated T lymphocytes, induced production of interleukine-10 and decreased collagenase activity (11).

Recent research has highlighted the fact that, in atopic dermatitis (mild and moderate forms), the application of narrow-band UVB phototherapy (311-313 nm) is as efficient as UVA therapy, the duration of irradiation and the calorigenic effect being reduced (12). The same form of NB-UVB was successfully applied to the treatment of psoriasis (13), lichen planus (14), vitiligo (15) and pityriasis lichenoides (16). Research targeting the effects of ultraviolet radiation (PUVA and UVB) on allergic disorders found that: UV light inhibits sensitization to some contact allergens (haptens); after irradiation with UV light, the number of regulatory T cells increases; UV light inhibits histamine release from mast cells, thus diminishing the acute urticarial reaction (17).

c) visible and ultraviolet light combination

One of the most recent therapeutic successes of phototherapy comes from the idea of associating visible and ultraviolet light and applying this light to the inflamed nasal mucosa in cases of allergic rhinitis (18). This technique will be detailed in the following chapter.

Clinic Study

We conducted a multi-center study which included four study centers – Arad, Carei, Oradea, Timisoara – all equipped with the same devices: acoustic rhinomanometer and allergy-screen set for serological allergy dosage, each patient being subject to a study protocol which we shall present below.

Inclusion criteria

We have considered that the most important criteria for the inclusion of patients in the study are as follows:
- age ranging from 10 to 60 years
- cumulative symptomatic score: minimum 5
- positive allergy test
- the patient has given his written informed consent

Cumulative symptomatic score

Nasal obstruction
- 0 – absent
- 1 – 0 to 1 hour/12 hours
- 2 – 1 to 2 hours/12 hours
- 3 – >2 hours /12 hours

Sneezing
- 0 – absent
- 1 – <5 bouts/12 hours
- 2 – 5-10 bouts/12 hours
- 3 – >10 bouts/12 hours

Mucus production (rhinorrhea)
- 0 – absent
- 1 – present

General symptoms
- 0 – absent
- 1 – present

Posterior drainage of secretions
- 0 – absent
- 1 – present

Ocular symptoms (pruritus, lacrimation)
- 0 – absent
- 1 – present

Exclusion criteria

-   participation in another clinical study one month prior
-   a history of intolerance to medication used in the study
-   clinical symptoms of nasal and/or sinus infections
-   significant anatomic anomalies: nasal septum deviation, sub-septum deviation
-   nasal instillation with corticoids in the last two months
-   nasal polyps or a history of nasal polyps
-   other types of chronic rhinitis: chronic hypertrophic rhinitis, chronic drug-induced rhinitis
-   nasal surgical interventions six months prior
-   systemic administration of corticoids six months prior
-   pregnancy and nursing (for the drug treatment)
-   general administration of antihistamines one month prior
-   impossibility of communicating with the investigator
-   severe medical disorder
-   patients undergoing immunotherapy.

Study Protocol

Each patient who meets the inclusion criteria shall be subject to an examination protocol containing:

Case history
-   each patient shall state:
    o   personal data–full name, age , background (urban-rural)
    o   family and collateral history, insisting on allergic diseases, knowing that the likelihood of atopy in children is double when one parent is atopic, and when both parents are atopic, the risk increases four times
    o   personal pathological history - with an emphasis on other allergic diseases
    o   life and work conditions: exposure to occupational allergens, dietary habits, smoking, alcohol use

Objective ENT exam:

-   inspection and palpation
-   examination of the vestibule

- anterior rhinoscopy
- posterior rhinoscopy
- nasal and rhinopharyngeal endoscopy
- mouth and throat examination

Rhinomanometry

- it is preferable to use acoustic rhinomanometry, which is a speedy method with very good results in terms of nasal permeability and general consensus for the achievements of the method

Allergy test

- it involves skin testing (prick test) and serological allergy testing – see the annex on allergy testing

Investigation plan – visit schedule

1st VISIT
It will occur on the day of enrolment (day 1) or one day before:
- assessment of inclusion/exclusion criteria
- signing of the written consent by the patient
- establishment of the cumulative symptomatic score
- objective clinical ENT examination
- allergy testing
- rhinomanometry

2nd VISIT

It will occur between the 7th and 10th days of the study
- cumulative symptomatic score
- objective clinical ENT examination, not including endoscopy
- rhinomanometry

3rd VISIT

It will occur on the 14th day, including:
- cumulative symptomatic score

- objective clinical ENT examination
- rhinomanometry

4th VISIT

It will occur on the 27th-30th day and comprises the same examinations

5th VISIT (FOLLOW-UP)

It occurs on the 45th day and comprises:
- cumulative symptomatic score
- objective clinical ENT examination   -   rhinomanometry

The initial group included 187 patients, 90 of which were excluded after applying inclusion and exclusion criteria, the remaining 97 patients, which formed the actual study group, being randomized at a 2/1 ratio between phototherapy and placebo treatment.

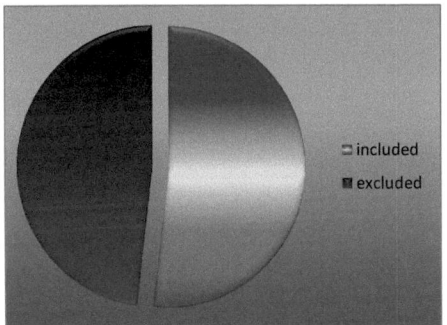

In this group, 60 patients were males, accounting for 62%, and 37 were females, accounting for 38% of the total.
Group distribution according to gender

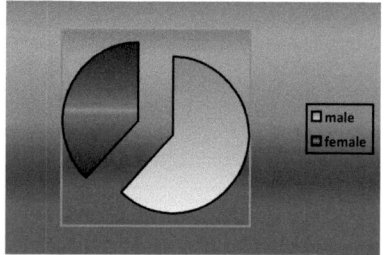

In terms of social background, most patients come from urban areas – 66 patients, accounting for 68%, and 31 patients hail from rural areas, accounting for the remaining 32%.

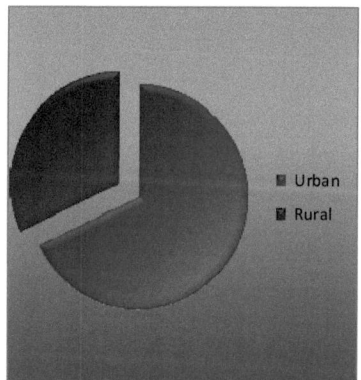

Group distribution according to social background

After obtaining the study group (97 patients), according to the criteria presented above, we conducted 2/1 randomization, that is, the first two patients were subject to phototherapy, whereas the following one received placebo treatment. Consequently, 65 patients received phototherapy, and 32 received placebo treatment.

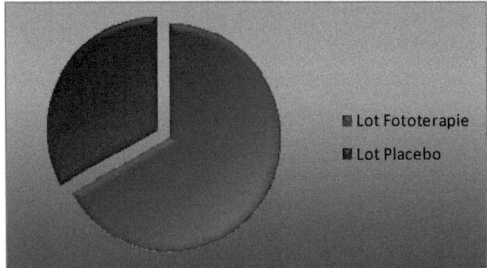

Patients treated with phototherapy/patients treated with placebo.

Patients were administered phototherapy using Rhinolight devices, manufactured by Rhinolight Ltd, Szeged, Hungary, three times a week, every other day, for two weeks, the sessions beginning at two minutes for each nostril, then increasing, by 15 seconds for each exposure, to three minutes, which were maintained in the last two sessions.

For patients who received the placebo treatment, a special filter was provided by the manufacturing company to stop the light.

Each patient received a self-evaluation form, which they completed on a daily basis, for the main symptoms of allergic rhinitis: nasal obstruction, rhinorrhea, sneezing, nasal pruritus, and ocular symptoms, on the following scale of severity: 0-absent, 1-mild, 2-moderate, 3-severe.

In parallel, the investigator assessed, during each visit, the state of the patient through case history and objective clinical examination, including endoscopy and acoustic rhinomanometry for an objective measurement of nasal obstruction.

Results

Patient assessment pursued several directions:
- the subjective assessment of each patient by symptoms
- the assessment of the cumulative symptomatic score by the examiner
- the examination of each separate symptom by the examiner
- the objective clinical examination completed by nasal endoscopy
- the measurement of air flow through acoustic rhinomanometry.

Of the 97 patients who took part in the study, 7 left the study, accounting for 7% of the total; among these, four were part of the control group who underwent placebo therapy.

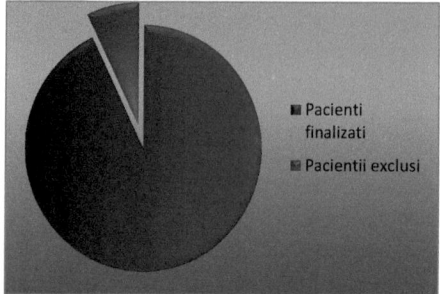

As regards the cumulative symptomatic score, it was calculated by the examiner at each separate visit and recorded in the patient's study sheet, the results being, of course, radically different for the two studied groups – phototherapy/placebo.

By reviewing the group of patients who underwent phototherapy, we noticed the following aspects: there were a number of 3 patients who left the study, accounting for 4.5% of the phototherapy group and 3 % of the total group, the most frequent cause being the inefficiency of the treatment.

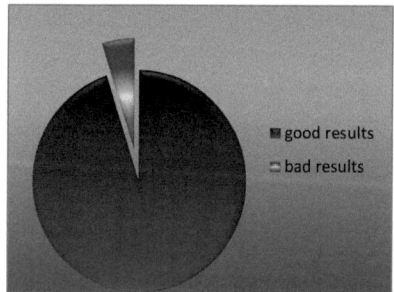

The evolution of the phototherapy group

Among the patients of this group, therapeutic results were good; the examiners quantified this positive result, this state of well-being into very good improvement – 43 patients, equivalent to 67%, and good improvement – 19 patients, accounting for a percentage of 28 % of the total.

By comparing the cumulative symptomatic score calculated by each examiner at each visit to the subjective one established by each patient before the phototherapy session, we noted a general agreement between the two criteria, the difference usually favoring the cumulative symptomatic score, but without statistically significant differences.

By studying the relation between the evolution of the cumulative symptomatic score and the results of rhinomanometry, we notice a general agreement; however, there is a difference of subjective perception of nasal obstruction in a percentage of 7% of the patients, where acoustic rhinomanometry showed an evident improvement, whereas the subjective sensation of these patients was greatly diminished.

Overall, there was a correlation between the evolution of the cumulative symptomatic score and the objective clinical examination of each patient.

By examining the placebo group, we noted the following results: very good in 3 patients – 10%, moderate improvement in 14 patients – 43% and unfavorable evolution in 15 patients – 47%.

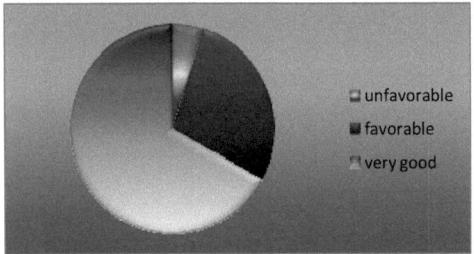

By comparing the two groups – phototherapy and placebo – we noted a very large difference in favor of the phototherapy group in view of its very good evolution – 43 patients/3 patients.

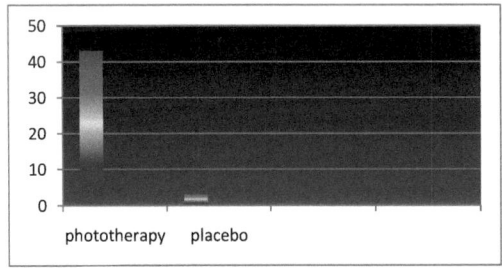

By comparing the percentages of patients with unfavorable evolution, we found that, within the placebo group, such patients are prevalent.

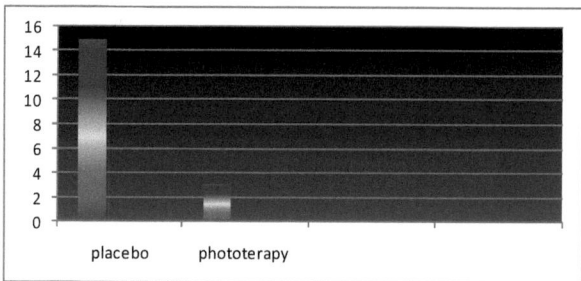

Patients with unfavorable evolution

Continuing the comparative statistical analysis, we find a relatively large proportion of moderate improvement for patients in the placebo group, this percentage being also influenced by the size of the patient group.

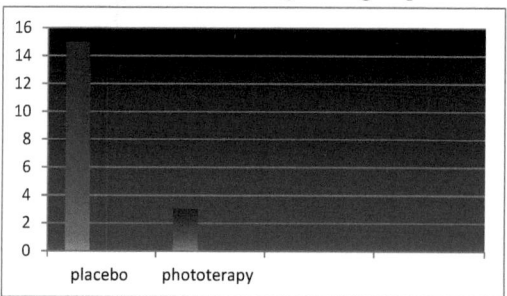

Patients with moderate improvement

Side effects

The most frequent side effect is dryness in the nasal mucosa, found in about 40% of the patients, a side effect which can be easily controlled by administering moisturizing solutions, in our case oily Vitamin A solution. Another rarer side effect was moderate epistaxis, present in 7 patients, accounting for 7% of the phototherapy group.

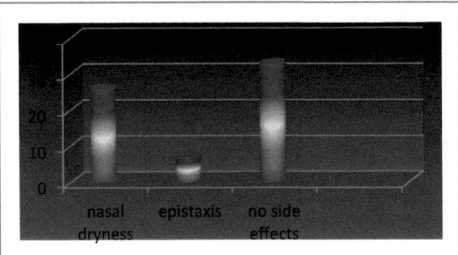

Conclusions

To conclude, we wish to review the most important objectives and rationales of the study of rhinophototherapy as an alternative method to the classic treatment of allergic rhinitis:

  - the main objective is to study phototherapy in the treatment of allergic rhinitis, as compared to classic drug treatment and placebo therapy

  - allergic rhinitis has become a global health issue, given the disease frequency in about 1,000,000 Romanian and Hungarian inhabitants in the studied area

  - healthcare costs for these patients are very high, which is why it is important to find a method that is efficient, while also being less expensive

  - drug therapy for allergic rhinitis has a high rate of failure

  - allergic rhinitis is not a life-threatening disease, but it is frequently associated with numerous diseases whose onset it can favor: asthma, rhino-sinusitis, otitis media, repeated infections of the lower airways

  - allergic rhinitis affects the patients' quality of life, their social life, academic performance and work productivity

  - through our joint effort, we wish to discover an efficient, secure therapeutic method, with no notable side effects, inexpensive, which would improve the health of our patients, Romanian and Hungarian alike, as well as their quality of life, since disease knows no boundaries and no differences among us.

  The conclusion of our study is that mUV/VIS phototherapy treatment (a combination of ultraviolet B rays - 5%, ultraviolet A rays -25% and low-intensity visible light) is efficient in treating allergic rhinitis, significantly improving the disease symptoms, as well as the total nasal symptomatic score.

  The treatment was well tolerated, the only side effect shown by the majority of patients being dryness of the nasal mucosa, which is easily controlled by intranasal administration of oily solutions.

  Phototherapy has no contraindications; it can be used in children, pregnant women, or athletes.

It can be stated with certainty that phototherapy is an alternative method of treatment to local and/or general classic drug treatment, being even indicated for patients where classic treatment has failed, and we, ENT and allergology practitioners, know that these cases have occurred with increased frequency in recent times. To this end we seek to extend our study further by gathering a group of patients who showed no results after classic treatment, to whom we will administer phototherapy.

As such, we can assert, by analyzing the study's preliminary data, that phototherapy is efficient as a therapeutic method in treating patients with allergic rhinitis, being also well-tolerated, with only minor side effects that are easy to monitor and treat

Rhinophototherapy with RhinoLight

RhinoLight is listed among the attempts for nasal phototherapy, being based on the immunosuppressive and anti-inflammatory effect of UVA and UVB electromagnetic radiation.
It was conceived and developed by experts in optics and quantum mechanics, as well as dermatology and allergic diseases, from the University of Szeged (Hungary)
RhinoLight treatment consists of controlled exposure of the nasal mucosa to high-intensity cold light with a special, patented composition which has not been used in other rhinophototherapy attempts. ([1,2,3 and 4])
The spectrum of radiation used in RhinoLight treatment comprises 70% visible light, 25% ultraviolet A (UVA) radiation, and under 5% ultraviolet B (UVB) radiation.
Studies have shown that the exposure of the nasal mucosa to RhinoLight has the following physio-pathological effects ([5,6,7,8 and 9]):
1. it blocks histamine release from mast cells
2. it blocks allergen-induced histamin release
3. it induces apoptosis in T lymphocytes and eosinophils
4. it reduces ECP and interleukin 5 levels, as well as the number of eosinophils in nasal secretions, which are regarded as markers of allergic inflammation.

The practice of RhinoLight therapy

RhinLight treatment is indicated in seasonal or perennial allergic rhinitis, either alone or in combination with antihistamines or nasal corticotherapy.

A relative contraindication of the treatment is represented by severe anatomical changes of the nasal cavity, tumors, and infections. ENT assessment is essential before commencing the treatment.

A protocol has been proposed for applying the RhinoLight treatment to seasonal allergic rhinitis, consisting of several treatment sessions with a progressive increase in the duration of exposure, according to the following scheme:

Treatment session	Duration of treatment per nostril in minutes: seconds
First week	
1	2:00
2	2:15
3	2:30
Second week	
4	2:45
5	3:00
6	3:00

In the case of perennial rhinitis, the recommended therapeutic protocol is:

Treatment session	Duration of treatment per nostril in minutes: seconds
First week	
1	2:00
2	2:15
3	2:30
Second week	
4	2:45
Third week	
5	3:00
Fourth week	

6	3:00
Fifth week	
7	3:00
Sixth week	
8	3:00

It is recommended, on the one hand, that the duration of exposure does not exceed 3 minutes, and on the other hand, to avoid administering more than four treatment sessions per week.

Efficiency of RhinoLight therapy

The studies conducted so far have revealed the favorable effect of RhinoLight in the treatment of seasonal and perennial allergic rhinitis.

Koreck et al ([1]) found an important and statistically significant improvement in the total symptomatic score, as compared to placebo, in patients with allergic rhinitis in a double-blind randomized and placebo-controlled study. A significant improvement was noted in all symptom scores for nasal obstruction, rhinorrhea, sneezing and nasal pruritus.

Koreck et al also compared, in an open study, the efficiency of RhinoLight treatment to the 180 mg/day p.o. fexofenadine treatment. The results showed the superior efficiency of this method of rhinophototherapy.

Safety of RhinoLight therapy

Due to its special composition, it is believed that this treatment method does not induce heat production in the mucosa, being thus painless. Clinical studies have demonstrated that no irreversible or malignant lesions occur in exposed tissues.

Bibliography

1. Andrea I Koreck, Zsanett Csoma, Laszlo Bodai, Ferenc Ignacz, Anna Sz. Kenderessy, Edit Kadocsa, Gabor Szabo, Zsolt Bor, Anna Erdei, Barnabas Szony, Bernhard Homey, Attila Dobozy, Lajos Kemeny: Rhinophototherapy: a new therapeutic tool for the management of allergic rhinitis. J Allergy Clin Immunol, March 2005, Vol. 115, Number 3: 541-47

2. Koreck A, Csoma Zs, Ignácz F, Bodai L, Kadocsa E, Szabó G, Bor Zs, Nékám K, Dobozy A, Kemény L: Intranasalis fototerápia az allergiás rhinitis kezelésében (Intranasal phototherapy for the treatment of allergic rhinitis). Orv. Hetil. 2005, 146(19): 965-969

3. G. Passalacqua, P. J. Bousquet, Kai-H. Carlsen, J. Kemp, R. F. Lockey, B. Niggemann, R. Pawankar, D. Price, J. Bousquet: ARIA update – Systematic review of complementary and alternative medicine for rhinitis and asthma. J Allergy Clin Immunol, May 2006, Vol. 117, Number 5: 1054-1062

4. Kadocsa E, Koreck I. A, Bella Zs, Csoma Zs, Ignácz F, Alexa M, Dobozy A, Jóri J, Kemény L: Intranasalis fototerápia: új terápiás eljárás allergiás rhinitisben. (Intranasal phototherapy: new therapeutical method in the treatment of allergic rhinitis) Fül-, orr-, gégegyógyászat 2006, 52(2): 108-114

5. Csoma Zs, Ignacz F, Bor Zs, Szabo G, Bodai L, Dobozy A, Kemeny L: Intranasal irradiation with the xenon chloride ultraviolet B laser improves allergic rhinitis. J Photochem Photobiol B: Biology, 2004, 75, Issue 3: 137-44

6. Koreck A, Csoma Zs, Ignacz F, Bodai L, Dobozy A, Kemeny L: Inhibition of immediate type hypersensitivity reaction by combined irradiation with ultraviolet and visible light. J Photochem Photobiol B: Biology, 2004, 77: 93-96

7. Kronauer C, Eberlein-Konig B, Ring J, Behrendt H: Influence of UVB, UVA and UVA1 irradiation on histamine release from human basophils and mast cells in vitro in the presence and absence of antioxidants. Photochem Photobiol, 2003; 77: 531-4

8. Z Novák, A Bérces, Gy Rontó, É Pállinger, A Dobozy, L Kemény: Efficacy of different UV-emitting light sources in the induction of T-cell apoptosis. J Photchem Photobiol, 2004, 79(5): 434-439

9. Zsanett Csoma, Andrea Koreck, Ferenc Ignacz, Zsolt Bor, Gabor Szabo, Laszlo Bodai, Attila Dobozy and Lajos Kemeny: PUVA treatment of the nasal cavity improves the clinical symptoms of allergic rhinitis and inhibits the immediate-

type hypersensitivity reaction in the skin. Journal of Photochemistry and Photobiology B: Biology 83 (2006) 21-26

10. Lajos Kemény, Andrea Koreck: Ultraviolet light phototherapy for allergic rhinitis. Review in the Journal of Photochemistry and Photobiology B: Biology 87 (2007) 58–65
11. L. Kemény, A. Koreck, A. Szechenyi, M. Morocz, A. Cimpean, Zs. Bella, E. Garaczi M. Raica, T.R. Olariu, I. Rasko: Effects of intranasal phototherapy on nasal mucosa in patients with allergic rhinitis. Journal of Photochemistry and Photobiology B: Biology 89 (2007) 163–169

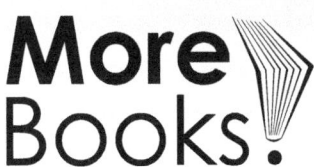
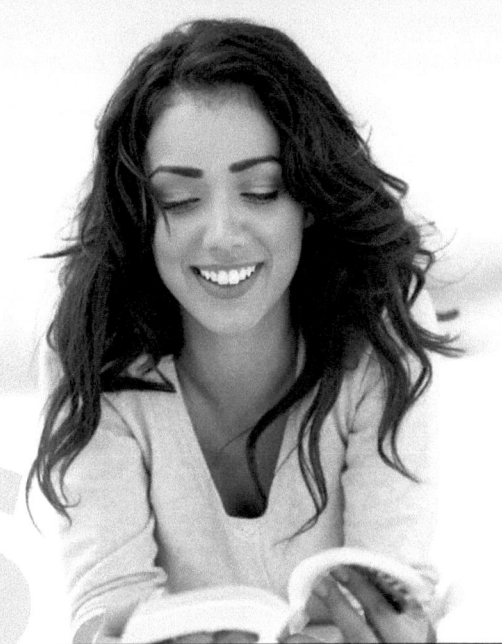

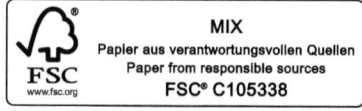
Printed by Books on Demand GmbH, Norderstedt / Germany